My Air Fryer Toaster Oven Cookbook

Easy & Healthy Air Fryer Toaster Oven Recipes To Make Unforgettable First Courses

Eva Morris

TABLE OF CONTENT

medical or professional advice. The content within this book has been derived from various sources. Please consult a licensed professional before attempting any techniques outlined in this book.

By reading this document, the reader agrees that under no circumstances is the author responsible for any losses, direct or indirect, which are incurred as a result of the use of information contained within this document, including, but not limited to, — errors, omissions, or inaccuracies.

Chocolate Bites

Preparation Time: 15 minutes

Cooking Time: 13 minutes

Servings: 8

Ingredients:

- 2 cups plain flour
- Two tablespoons cocoa powder
- ½ cup icing sugar
- Pinch of ground cinnamon
- One teaspoon vanilla extract
- ¾ cup chilled butter
- ¼ cup chocolate, chopped into eight chunks

Directions:

1. In a bowl, mix the flour, icing sugar, cocoa powder, cinnamon, and vanilla extract.

2. With a pastry cutter, cut the butter and mix till a smooth dough forms.

3. Divide the dough into eight equal-sized balls.

4. Press one chocolate chunk in the center of each ball and cover with the dough thoroughly.

5. Place the balls into the baking pan.

6. Press "Power Button" of Air Fry Oven and turn the dial to select the "Air Fry" mode.

7. Press the Time button and again turn the dial to set the cooking time to 8 minutes.

8. Now push the Temp button and rotate the dial to set the temperature at 355 degrees F.

9. Press the "Start/Pause" button to start.

10. When the unit beeps to show that it is preheated, open the lid.

11. Arrange the pan in "Air Fry Basket" and insert it in the oven.

12. After 8 minutes of cooking, set the temperature at 320 degrees F for 5 minutes.

13. Place the baking pan onto the wire rack to cool completely before serving.

Nutrition:

Calories 328

Total Fat 19.3 g

Saturated Fat 12.2 g

Cholesterol 47 mg

Sodium 128 mg

Total Carbs 35.3 g

Fiber 1.4 g

Sugar 10.2 g

Protein 4.1 g

Shortbread Fingers

Preparation Time: 15 minutes

Cooking Time: 12 minutes

Servings: 10

Ingredients:

- 1/3 cup caster sugar
- 1 2/3 cups plain flour
- ¾ cup butter

Directions:

1. In a large bowl, mix the sugar and flour.

2. Add the butter and mix until a smooth dough forms.

3. Cut the dough into ten equal-sized fingers.

4. With a fork, lightly prick the fingers.

5. Place the fingers into the lightly greased baking pan.

6. Press "Power Button" of Air Fry Oven and turn the dial to select the "Air Fry" mode.

7. Press the Time button and again turn the dial to set the cooking time to 12 minutes.

8. Now push the Temp button and rotate the dial to set the temperature at 355 degrees F.

9. Press the "Start/Pause" button to start.

10. When the unit beeps to show that it is preheated, open the lid.

11. Arrange the pan in "Air Fry Basket" and insert it in the oven.

12. Place the baking pan onto a wire rack to cool for about 5-10 minutes.

13. Now, invert the shortbread fingers onto a wire rack to completely cool before serving.

Nutrition:

Calories 223

Total Fat 14 g

Saturated Fat 8.8 g

Cholesterol 37 mg

Sodium 99 mg

Total Carbs 22.6 g

Fiber 0.6 g

Sugar 0.7 g

Protein 2.3 g

Berry Tacos

Preparation Time: 15 minutes

Cooking Time: 5 minutes

Servings: 2

Ingredients:

- Two soft shell tortillas
- Four tablespoons strawberry jelly
- ¼ cup fresh blueberries
- ¼ cup fresh raspberries
- Two tablespoons powdered sugar

Directions:

1. Spread two tablespoons of strawberry jelly over each tortilla
2. Top each with berries evenly and sprinkle with powdered sugar.
3. Press "Power Button" of Air Fry Oven and turn the dial to select the "Air Fry" mode.
4. Press the Time button and again turn the dial to set the cooking time to 5 minutes.

5. Now push the Temp button and rotate the dial to set the temperature at 300 degrees F.

6. Press the "Start/Pause" button to start.

7. When the unit beeps to show that it is preheated, open the lid.

8. Arrange the tortillas in "Air Fry Basket" and insert it in the oven.

9. Serve warm.

Nutrition:

Calories 216

Total Fat 0.8 g

Saturated Fat 0.1 g

Cholesterol 0mg

Sodium 11 mg

Total Carbs 53.2 g

Fiber 3 g

Sugar 38.7 g

Protein 1.7 g

Apple Pastries

Preparation Time: 15 minutes

Cooking Time: 10 minutes

Servings: 6

Ingredients:

- ½ of a large apple, peeled, cored, and chopped

- One teaspoon fresh orange zest, grated finely

- ½ tablespoon white sugar

- ½ teaspoon ground cinnamon

- 7.05oz. prepared frozen puff pastry

Directions:

1. In a bowl, mix all ingredients except puff pastry.

2. Cut the pastry into 16 squares.

3. Place about a teaspoon of the apple mixture in the center of each square.

4. Fold each square into a triangle and press the edges slightly with wet fingers.

5. Then with a fork, press the edges firmly.

6. Press "Power Button" of Air Fry Oven and turn the dial to select the "Air Fry" mode.

7. Press the Time button and again turn the dial to set the cooking time to 10 minutes.

8. Now push the Temp button and rotate the dial to set the temperature at 390 degrees F.

9. Press the "Start/Pause" button to start.

10. When the unit beeps to show that it is preheated, open the lid.

11. Arrange the pastries in a greased "Air Fry Basket" and insert it in the oven.

12. Serve warm.

Nutrition:

Calories 198

Total Fat 12.7 g

Saturated Fat 3.2 g

Cholesterol 0 mg

Sodium 83 mg

Total Carbs 18.8 g

Fiber 1.1 g

Sugar 3.2 g

Protein 2.5 g

Perfect Cinnamon Toast

Preparation Time: 10 minutes

Cooking time: 5 minutes

Servings: 6

Ingredients

- 2 tsp. pepper
- 1½ tsp. vanilla extract
- 1½ tsp. cinnamon
- ½ C. sweetener of choice
- 1C. coconut oil
- 12 slices whole-wheat bread

Directions:

1. Melt coconut oil and mix with sweetener until dissolved. Mix in remaining ingredients minus bread till incorporated.

2. Spread mixture onto bread, covering all areas.

3. Pour the coated pieces of bread into the Oven rack/basket. Place the Rack on the

middle-shelf of the Air fryer oven. Set temperature to 400°F, and set time to 5 minutes.

4. Remove and cut diagonally. Enjoy!

Nutrition: CALORIES: 124; FAT: 2G; PROTEIN: 0G; SUGAR: 4G

Easy Baked Chocolate Mug Cake

Preparation Time: 5 minutes

Cooking time: 15 minutes

Servings: 3

Ingredients

- ½ cup cocoa powder

- ½ cup stevia powder

- 1cup coconut cream

- 1package cream cheese, room temperature

- 1tablespoon vanilla extract

- 1tablespoons butter

Directions:

1. Preheat the air fryer oven for 5 minutes.

2. In a mixing bowl, combine all ingredients.

3. Use a hand mixer to mix everything until fluffy.

4. Pour into greased mugs.

5. Place the mugs in the fryer basket.

6. Bake for 15 minutes at 350°F.

7. Place in the fridge to chill before serving.

Nutrition: CALORIES: 744; FAT: 69.7G; PROTEIN:13.9G; SUGAR:4G

Angel Food Cake

Preparation Time: 5minutes

Cooking Time: 30minutes

Serving: 4

Ingredients

- ¼ cup butter, melted
- 1cup powdered erythritol
- 1teaspoon strawberry extract
- 12 egg whites
- 2teaspoons cream of tartar
- A pinch of salt

Directions:

1. Preheat the air fryer oven for 5 minutes.
2. Mix the egg whites and cream of tartar.
3. Use a hand mixer and whisk until white and fluffy.
4. Add the rest of the ingredients except for the butter and whisk for another minute.
5. Pour into a baking dish.

6. Place in the air fryer basket and cook for 30 minutes at 400°F or if a toothpick inserted in the middle comes out clean.

7. Drizzle with melted butter once cooled.

Nutrition: CALORIES: 65; FAT: 5G; PROTEIN: 3.1G; FIBER: 1G

Fried Peaches

Preparation Time: 130 minutes

Cooking Time: 15 minutes

Serving: 4

Ingredients

- 4ripe peaches (1/2 a peach = 1 serving)
- 1 1/2 cups flour
- **Salt**
- **2egg yolks**
- 3/4 cups cold water
- 11/2 tablespoons olive oil
- 2tablespoons brandy
- **4egg whites**
- Cinnamon/sugar mix

Directions:

1. Combine flour, egg yolks, and salt in a mixing bowl. Slowly mix in water, and

then add brandy. Set the mixture aside for 2 hours and do something for 1 hour 45 minutes.

2. Boil a large pot of water and cut and X at the bottom of each peach. While the water boils, fill another large bowl with water and ice. Boil each peach for about a minute, and then plunge it in the ice bath. Now the peels should fall off the peach. Beat the egg whites and mix into the butter mix. Dip each peach in the mixture to coat.

3. Pour the coated peach into the Oven rack/basket. Place the Rack on the middle-shelf of the Air fryer oven. Set temperature to 360°F, and set time to 10 minutes.

4. Prepare a plate with cinnamon/sugar mix, roll peaches in the mixture and serve.

Nutrition: CALORIES: 306; FAT: 3G; PROTEIN: 10G; FIBER: 2.7G

Apple Dumplings

Preparation Time: 10 minutes

Cooking Time: 25 minutes

Serving: 4

Ingredients

- 2tbsp. melted coconut oil
- 2puff pastry sheets
- 1tbsp. brown sugar
- 2tbsp. raisins
- 2small apples of choice

Directions:

1. Ensure your air fryer oven is preheated to 356 degrees.

2. Core and peel apples and mix with raisins and sugar.

3. Place a bit of apple mixture into puff pastry sheets and brush sides with melted coconut oil.

4. Place into the air fryer. Cook 25 minutes, we were turning halfway through. It will be

golden when done.

Nutrition: CALORIES: 367; FAT: 7G; PROTEIN: 2G; SUGAR: 5G

Apple Pie In Air Fryer

Preparation Time: 5 minutes

Cooking Time: 35 minutes

Serving: 4

Ingredients

- ½ teaspoon vanilla extract
- 1beaten egg
- 1large apple, chopped
- 1Pillsbury Refrigerator pie crust
- 1tablespoon butter
- 1tablespoon ground cinnamon
- 1tablespoon raw sugar
- 2tablespoon sugar
- 2teaspoons lemon juice
- Baking spray

Directions:

1. Lightly grease baking pan of air fryer oven with cooking spray. Spread the pie crust on the bottom of the pan up to the sides.

2. In a bowl, mix vanilla, sugar, cinnamon, lemon juice, and apples. Pour on top of pie crust.

3. Top apples with butter slices.

4. Cover apples with the other pie crust. Pierce with the knife the tops of the pie.

5. Spread beaten egg on top of crust and sprinkle sugar.

6. Cover with foil.

7. For 25 minutes, cook at 390°F.

8. Remove foil cook for 10 minutes at 330oF until tops are browned.

9. Serve and enjoy.

Nutrition: CALORIES: 372; FAT: 19G; PROTEIN: 4.2G; SUGAR: 5G

Air Fryer Chocolate Cake

Preparation Time: 5 minutes

Cooking Time: 35 minutes

Serving: 9

Ingredients

- ½ C. hot water

- 1tsp. vanilla

- ¼ C. olive oil

- ½ C. almond milk

- 1egg

- ½ tsp. Salt

- ¾ tsp. Baking soda

- ¾ tsp. baking powder

- ½ C. unsweetened cocoa powder

- 2C. almond flour

- 1C. brown sugar

Directions:

1. Preheat your air fryer oven to 356 degrees.

2. Stir all dry ingredients together. Then stir in wet ingredients. Add hot water last.

3. The batter will be thin, no worries.

4. Pour cake batter into a pan that fits into the fryer. Cover with foil and poke holes into the foil.

5. Bake 35 minutes.

6. Discard foil and then bake another 10 minutes.

Nutrition: CALORIES: 378; FAT: 9G; PROTEIN: 4G; SUGAR: 5G

Banana-Choco Brownies

Preparation Time: 5 minutes

Cooking Time: 30 minutes

Serving: 12

Ingredients

- 2cups almond flour
- 2teaspoons baking powder
- ½ teaspoon baking powder
- ½ teaspoon baking soda
- ½ teaspoon salt
- 1over-ripe banana
- 3large eggs
- ½ teaspoon stevia powder
- ¼ cup of coconut oil
- 1tablespoon vinegar
- 1/3 cup almond flour
- 1/3 cup cocoa powder

Directions:

1. Preheat the air fryer oven for 5 minutes.

2. Combine all ingredients in a food processor and pulse until well-combined.

3. Pour into a baking dish that will fit in the air fryer.

4. Place in the air fryer basket and cook for 30 minutes at 350°F or if a toothpick inserted in the middle comes out clean.

Nutrition: CALORIES: 75; FAT: 6.5G; PROTEIN: 1.7G; SUGAR: 2G

Chocolate Donuts

Preparation Time: 5 minutes

Cooking Time: 20 minutes

Serving: 8-10

Ingredients

- (8-ounce) can jumbo biscuits

- Cooking oil

- Chocolate sauce, such as Hershey's

Directions:

1. Separate the biscuit dough into eight biscuits and place them on a flat work surface. Use a small circle cookie cutter or a biscuit cutter to cut a hole in each biscuit center. You can also cut the holes using a knife.

2. Spray the air fryer basket with cooking oil.

3. Place four donuts in the air fryer oven. Do not stack. Spray with cooking oil. Set temperature to 350°F. Cook for 4 minutes.

4. Open the air fryer and flip the donuts—Cook for an additional 4 minutes.

5. Remove the cooked donuts from the air fryer oven, and then repeat for the remaining four donuts.

6. Drizzle chocolate sauce over the donuts and enjoy while warm.

Nutrition: CALORIES: 181; FAT: 98G; PROTEIN: 3G; FIBER: 1G

Easy Air Fryer Donuts

Preparation Time: 5 minutes

Cooking Time: 5 minutes

Serving: 8

Ingredients

- Pinch of allspice
- 4tbsp. dark brown sugar
- ½ - 1 tsp. cinnamon
- 1/3 C. granulated sweetener
- 3tbsp. melted coconut oil
- 1can of biscuits

Directions:

1. Mix allspice, sugar, sweetener, and cinnamon.

2. Take out biscuits from can and with a circle cookie cutter, cut holes from centers, and place into the air fryer.

3. Cook 5 minutes at 350 degrees. As batches are cooked, use a brush to coat with melted coconut oil and dip each into sugar

mixture.

4. Serve warm!

Nutrition: CALORIES: 209; FAT: 4G; PROTEIN: 0G;
SUGAR: 3G

Chocolate Soufflé For Two

Preparation Time: 5minutes

Cooking Time: 14 minutes

Serving: 2

Ingredients

- 2tbsp. Almond flour
- ½ tsp. vanilla
- 3tbsp. sweetener
- 2separated eggs
- ¼ C. melted coconut oil
- 3ounces of semi-sweet chocolate, chopped

Directions:

1. Brush coconut oil and sweetener onto ramekins.

2. Melt coconut oil and chocolate together.

3. Beat egg yolks well, adding vanilla and sweetener. Stir in flour and ensure there are no lumps.

4. Preheat the air fryer oven to 330 degrees.

5. Whisk egg whites till they reach peak state and fold them into chocolate mixture.

6. Pour batter into ramekins and place them into the air fryer oven.

7. Cook 14 minutes.

8. Serve with powdered sugar dusted on top.

Nutrition: CALORIES: 238; FAT: 6G; PROTEIN: 1G; SUGAR: 4G

Fried Bananas With Chocolate Sauce

Preparation Time: 10 minutes

Cooking Time: 10 minutes

Serving: 2

Ingredients

- 1large egg
- ¼ cup cornstarch
- ¼ cup plain bread crumbs
- 3bananas halved crosswise
- Cooking oil
- Chocolate sauce (see

Ingredient tip)

Directions:

1. In a small bowl, beat the egg. In another bowl, place the cornstarch.
2. Place the breadcrumbs in a third bowl.

3. Dip the bananas in the cornstarch, then the egg, and then the breadcrumbs.

4. Spray the air fryer basket with cooking oil. Place the bananas in the basket and spray them with cooking oil.

5. Set temperature to 360°F and cook for 5 minutes. Open the air fryer and flip the bananas—Cook for an additional 2 minutes. Transfer the bananas to plates.

6. Drizzle the chocolate sauce over the bananas and serve.

7. You can make your chocolate sauce using two tablespoons of milk and ¼ cup chocolate chips. Heat a saucepan over medium-high heat. Add the milk and stir for 1 to 2 minutes. Add the chocolate chips. Stir for 2 minutes, or until the chocolate has melted.

Nutrition: CALORIES: 203; FAT: 6G; PROTEIN: 3G; FIBER: 3G

Apple Hand Pies

Preparation Time: 5 minutes

Cooking Time: 8 minutes

Serving: 6

Ingredients

- 15-ounces no-sugar-added apple pie filling
- 1store-bought crust

Directions:

1. Layout the pie crust and slice it into equal-sized squares.

2. Place 2 tbsp. We are filling into each square and seal the crust with a fork.

3. Pour into the Oven rack/basket. Place the Rack on the middle-shelf of the Air fryer oven. Set temperature to 390°F, and set time to 8 minutes until golden in color.

Nutrition: CALORIES: 278; FAT: 10G; PROTEIN: 5G; SUGAR: 4G

Chocolaty Banana Muffins

Preparation Time: 5 minutes

Cooking Time: 25 minutes

Serving: 12

Ingredients

- ¾ cup whole wheat flour
- ¾ cup plain flour
- ¼ cup of cocoa powder
- ¼ teaspoon baking powder
- 1teaspoon baking soda
- ¼ teaspoon salt
- 2large bananas, peeled and mashed
- 1cup sugar
- 1/3 cup canola oil
- 1egg
- ½ teaspoon vanilla essence
- 1cup mini chocolate chips

Directions:

1. In a large bowl, mix flour, cocoa powder, baking powder, baking soda, and salt.

2. In another bowl, add bananas, sugar, oil, egg, and vanilla extract and beat till well combined.

3. Slowly, add flour mixture to egg mixture and mix till just combined.

4. Fold in chocolate chips.

5. Preheat the air fryer oven to 345 degrees F. Grease 12 muffin molds.

6. Transfer the mixture into prepared muffin molds evenly and cooks for about 20-25 minutes or till a toothpick inserted in the center comes out clean.

7. Remove the Air fryer's muffin molds and keep on a wire rack to cool for about 10 minutes. Carefully turn on a wire rack to cool completely before serving.

Air Fryer Apple Pies

Preparation Time: 10 minutes

Cooking Time: 25 minutes

Serving: 4

Ingredients

- 4tbsp butter

- 6tbsp brown sugar

- 1tsp ground cinnamon

- 2medium Granny Smith apples, diced

- 1tsp cornstarch

- 2tsp cold water

- 1/2 (14 oz.) package pastry to get a 9-inch double-crust pie

- cooking spray

- 1/2 tablespoon grapeseed oil

- 1/4 cup powdered sugar

- 1tsp milk, or more as required

Directions:

1. Combine apples, butter, brown sugar, and cinnamon in a skillet. Cook over moderate heat until apples have softened, about 5 minutes.

2. Dissolve cornstarch in cold water. Stir into apple mixture and cook until sauce thickens about 1 minute. Eliminate apple pie filling from heat and set aside to cool while you prepare the crust.

3. Unroll the pie crust onto a lightly floured surface and roll out slightly to smooth the dough's surface. Cut the dough into rectangles small enough so that two can fit on your air fryer simultaneously. Repeat with remaining crust until you've got eight equal rectangles, re-rolling a few of the bits of dough if necessary.

4. Wet the outer borders of 4 rectangles with water and then put some apple filling at the middle about 1/2-inch in the edges. Roll out the rest rectangles, so they are slightly more significant than the ones that

are served. Put these rectangles in addition to the filling; crimp the edges with a fork to seal. Cut four small slits from the tops of the pies.

5. Spray on the basket of an air fryer with cooking spray. Brush the tops of two tablespoons with grape seed oil and then move pies into the air fryer basket using a spatula.

6. Insert jar and then place the temperature to 385 degrees F (195 degrees C). Bake until golden brown, about 8 minutes. Remove pies in the basket and then repeat with the rest two pies.

7. Mix powdered milk and sugar in a small bowl. Brush glaze on hot pies and let to dry. Drink pops warm or at room temperature.

Beef Enchilada Dip

Preparation Time: 5 minutes

Cooking time: 10 minutes

Servings: 8

Ingredients:

- 2 lbs. ground beef
- ½ onion, chopped fine
- Two cloves garlic, chopped fine
- 2 cups enchilada sauce
- 2 cups Monterrey Jack cheese, grated
- 2 tbsp. sour cream

Directions:

1. Place rack in position 1.

2. Heat a large skillet over med-high heat. Add beef and cook until it starts to brown. Drain off fat.

3. Stir in onion and garlic and cook until tender, about 3 minutes. Stir in enchilada sauce and transfer mixture to a small casserole dish and top with cheese.

4. Set oven to convection bake at 325°F for 10 minutes. After 5 minutes, add casserole to the range and bake 3-5 minutes until cheese is melted and the mixture is heated through.

5. Serve warm topped with sour cream.

Nutrition:

Calories 414, Total Fat 22g, Saturated Fat 10g, Total Carbs 15g, Net Carbs 11g, Protein 39g, Sugar 8g, Fiber 4g, Sodium 1155mg, Potassium 635mg, Phosphorus 385mg

Cheesy Stuffed Sliders

Preparation Time: 15minutes

Cooking time: 50 minutes

Servings: 10

Ingredients:

- 2 tbsp. garlic powder

- 1 ½ tsp. salt

- 2 tsp. pepper

- 2 lbs. ground beef

- 8 oz. mozzarella slices, cut into 20 small pieces

- 20 potato slider rolls

Directions:

1. Place the baking pan in position 2.

2. In a small bowl, combine garlic powder, salt, and pepper.

3. Use 1 ½ tablespoon ground beef per patty. Roll it into a ball and press an indentation in the ball with your thumb.

4. Place a piece of cheese into beef and fold over sides to cover it completely. Flatten to ½-inch thick by 3-inches wide. Season both sides with garlic mixture.

5. Place patties in the fryer basket in a single layer and place it on the baking pan. Set oven to air fry on 350°F for 10 minutes. Turn patties over halfway through cooking time. Repeat with any remaining patties.

6. Place patties on bottoms of rolls and top with your favorite toppings. Serve immediately.

Nutrition:

Calories 402, Total Fat 14g, Saturated Fat 5g, Total Carbs 31g, Net Carbs 29g, Protein 38g, Sugar 3g, Fiber 2g, Sodium 835mg, Potassium 397mg, Phosphorus 400mg

Philly Egg Rolls

Preparation Time: 10 minutes

Cooking time: 25 minutes

Servings: 6

Ingredients:

- Nonstick cooking spray
- ½ lb. lean ground beef
- ¼ tsp. Garlic powder
- ¼ tsp. Onion powder
- ¼ tsp. Salt
- ¼ tsp. pepper
- ¾ cup green bell pepper, chopped
- ¾ cup onion, chopped
- Two slices of provolone cheese, torn into pieces
- 3 tbsp. cream cheese
- 6 square egg roll wrappers

Directions:

1. Place the baking pan in position 2. Lightly spray fryer basket with cooking spray.

2. Heat a large skillet over med-high heat.
   Add beef, garlic powder, onion powder,
   salt, and pepper. Stir to combine.

3. Add in bell pepper and onion and cook,
   occasionally stirring, until beef is no longer
   pink and vegetables are tender, about 6-8
   minutes.

4. Remove from heat and drain fat. Add
   provolone and cream cheese and stir until
   melted and combined. Transfer to a large
   bowl.

5. Lay egg roll wrappers, one at a time, on a
   dry work surface. Spoon about 1/3 cup
   mixture in a row just below the center of
   the wrapper. Moisten edges with water.
   Fold the sides in towards the middle and
   roll up around filling.

6. Place egg rolls, seam side down in fryer
   basket. Spray lightly with cooking spray.
   Place the basket in the oven and set it to
   air fry at 400°F for 10 minutes. Cook until
   golden brown, turning over halfway

through cooking time. Serve immediately.

Nutrition:

Calories 238, Total Fat 10g, Saturated Fat 5g, Total Carbs 21g, Net Carbs 20g, Protein 16g, Sugar 1g, Fiber 1g, Sodium 412mg, Potassium 206mg, Phosphorus 160mg

Mozzarella Cheese Sticks

Preparation Time: 10 minutes

Cooking time: 10minutes

Servings: 6

Ingredients:

- Nonstick cooking spray

- 12 Mozzarella cheese sticks, halved

- Two eggs

- ½ cup flour

- 1 ½ cups Italian panko bread crumbs

- ½ cup marinara sauce

Directions:

1. Blot cheese sticks with paper towels to soak up excess moisture.

2. In a shallow dish, beat eggs.

3. Place flour in a separate shallow dish.

4. Place bread crumbs in a third shallow dish.

5. Line a baking sheet with parchment paper.

6. One at a time, dip cheese sticks in egg, then flour, back in the egg, and finally in

bread crumbs. Place on prepared pan. Freeze 1-2 hours until completely frozen.

7. Place the baking pan in position 2 of the oven. Lightly spray fryer basket with cooking spray.

8. Place cheese sticks in a single layer in the basket and place it in the oven. Set to air fry on 375°F for 8 minutes. Cook until nicely browned and crispy, turning over halfway through cooking time. Serve with a marinara sauce for dipping.

Nutrition:

Calories 199, Total Fat 3g, Saturated Fat 1g, Total Carbs 30g, Net Carbs 28g, Protein 13g, Sugar 3g, Fiber 2g, Sodium 368mg, Potassium 175mg, Phosphorus 220mg

Buffalo Quesadillas

Preparation Time: 5 minutes

Cooking time: 5 minutes

Servings: 8

Ingredients:

- Nonstick cooking spray

- 2 cups chicken, cooked & chopped fine

- ½ cup Buffalo wing sauce

- 2 cups Monterey Jack cheese, grated

- ½ cup green onions, sliced thin

- Eight flour tortillas, 8-inch diameter

- ¼ cup blue cheese dressing

Directions:

1. Lightly spray the baking pan with cooking spray.

2. In a medium bowl, add chicken and wing sauce and toss to coat.

3. Place tortillas, one at a time, on the work surface. Spread ¼ of the chicken mixture over tortilla and sprinkle with cheese and

onion. Top with a second tortilla and place on the baking pan.

4. Set oven to broil at 400°F for 8 minutes. After 5 minutes, place the baking pan in position 2. Cook quesadillas 2-3 minutes per side until toasted and cheese has melted. Repeat with the remaining ingredients.

5. Cut quesadillas in wedges and serve with blue cheese dressing or other dipping sauce.

Nutrition:

Calories 376, Total Fat 20g, Saturated Fat 8g, Total Carbs 27g, Net Carbs 26g, Protein 22g, Sugar 2g, Fiber 2g, Sodium 685mg, Potassium 201mg, Phosphorus 301mg

Crispy Sausage Bites

Preparation Time: 5 minutes

Cooking time: 15 minutes

Servings: 12

Ingredients:

- Nonstick cooking spray
- 2 lbs. spicy pork sausage
- 1 ½ cups Bisques
- 4 cups sharp cheddar cheese, grated
- ½ cup onion diced fine
- 2 tsp. pepper
- 2 tsp. garlic, chopped fine

Directions:

1. Lightly spray the baking pan with cooking spray.

2. In a large bowl, combine all ingredients. Form into 1-inch balls and place them on the baking pan. These will need to be cooked in batches.

3. Set oven to bake at 375°F for 20 minutes. After 5 minutes, place baking pan in position two and cook 12-15 minutes or until golden brown. Repeat with remaining sausage bites. Serve immediately.

Nutrition

Calories 432, Total Fat 32g, Saturated Fat 13g, Total Carbs 14g, Net Carbs 14g, Protein 22g, Sugar 1g, Fiber 0g, Sodium 803mg, Potassium 286mg, Phosphorus 298mg

Puffed Asparagus Spears

Preparation Time: 20 minutes

Cooking time: 20 minutes

Servings: 10

Ingredients:

- Nonstick cooking spray

- 3 oz. prosciutto, sliced thin & cut into 30 long strips

- 30 asparagus spears, trimmed

- 10 (14 x 9-inch) sheets phyllo dough, thawed

Directions:

1. Place the baking pan in position 2 of the oven.

2. Wrap each asparagus spear with a piece of prosciutto, like a barber pole.

3. One at a time, place a sheet of phyllo on a work surface and cut into 3 4 1/2x9-inch rectangles.

4. Place an asparagus spear across a short end and roll-up—place in a single layer in

the fryer basket. Spray with cooking spray.

5. Place the basket in the oven and set it to air fry at 450°F for 10 minutes. Cook until phyllo is crisp and golden, about 8-10 minutes, turning over halfway through cooking time. Repeat with the remaining ingredients. Serve warm.

Nutrition

Calories 74, Total Fat 2g, Saturated Fat 0g, Total Carbs 11g, Net Carbs 10g, Protein 3g, Sugar 0g, Fiber 1g, Sodium 189mg, Potassium 60mg, Phosphorus 33mg

Wonton Poppers

Preparation Time: 15 minutes

Cooking time: 10 minutes

Servings: 10

Ingredients:

- Nonstick cooking spray

- One package refrigerated square wonton wrappers

- One 8-ounce package cream cheese softened

- Three jalapenos, seeds and ribs removed, finely chopped

- 1/2 cup shredded cheddar cheese

Directions:

1. Place the baking pan in position 2 of the oven. Lightly spray fryer basket with cooking spray.

2. In a large bowl, combine all ingredients except the wrappers until combined.

3. Put wrappers in a single layer on a baking sheet. Spoon a teaspoon of filling in the

center. Moisten the edges with water and fold wrappers over the filling, pinching edges to seal—place in a single layer in the basket.

4. Place the basket in the oven and set it to air fry at 375°F for 10 minutes. Cook until golden brown and crisp, turning over halfway through cooking time. Repeat with the remaining ingredients. Serve immediately.

Nutrition

Calories 287, Total Fat 11g, Saturated Fat 6g, Total Carbs 38g, Net Carbs 37g, Protein 9g, Sugar 1g, Fiber 1g, Sodium 485mg, Potassium 98mg, Phosphorus 104mg

Party Pull Apart

Preparation Time: 15minutes

Cooking time: 20 minutes

Servings: 10

Ingredients:

- Five cloves garlic
- 1/3 cup fresh parsley
- 2 tbsp. olive oil
- 4 oz. mozzarella cheese, sliced
- 3 tbsp. butter
- 1/8 tsp. salt
- One loaf sourdough bread

Directions:

1. Place the rack in position 1 of the oven.

2. In a food processor, add garlic, parsley, and oil and pulse until garlic is chopped fine.

3. Stack the mozzarella cheese and cut into 1 -inch squares.

4. Heat the butter in a small saucepan over medium heat. Add the garlic mixture and salt and cook 2 minutes, stirring occasionally. Remove from heat.

5. Use a sharp, serrated knife to make 1-inch diagonal cuts across the bread, being careful not to cut all the way through.

6. With a spoon, drizzle garlic butter into the cuts in the bread. Stack 3-4 cheese squares and place them in each of the cuts.

7. Place the bread on a sheet of foil and fold up the sides. Cut a second piece of foil just big enough to cover the top.

8. Set oven to convection bake at 350°F for 25 minutes. After 5 minutes, place the bread in the oven and bake for 10 minutes.

9. Remove the top piece of foil and bake 10 minutes more until the cheese has completely melted. Serve immediately.

Nutrition

Calories 173, Total Fat 7g, Saturated Fat 3g, Total Carbs 18g, Net Carbs 17g, Protein 7g, Sugar 2g, Fiber 1g,

Sodium 337mg, Potassium 68mg, Phosphorus 112mg

Easy Cheesy Stuffed Mushrooms

Preparation Time: 10 minutes

Cooking time: 15minutes

Servings: 4

Ingredients:

- Nonstick cooking spray
- 1/3 cup cream cheese, soft
- 1 tbsp. Parmesan cheese, grated
- ¼ tsp. garlic salt
- 2 tbsp. spinach, thaw, press dry & chop
- 8 oz. mushrooms, rinsed & stems removed
- 1 tbsp. panko bread crumbs

Directions:

1. Lightly spray the baking sheet with cooking spray.
2. In a medium bowl, combine cream cheese, parmesan, salt, and spinach; mix well.

3. Place mushrooms on the baking sheet and fill with cheese mixture. Sprinkle bread crumbs over the top.

4. Set an oven to bake at 350°F for 20 minutes. After 5 minutes, place the baking pan in position 2 of the range and cook mushrooms 15 minutes until tops are lightly browned. Serve hot.

Nutrition

Calories 121, Total Fat 7g, Saturated Fat 4g, Total Carbs 8g, Net Carbs 7g, Protein 4g, Sugar 2g, Fiber 1g, Sodium 168mg, Potassium 225mg, Phosphorus 86mg

Recipe Potato Chips Without Oil

Preparation Time: 10 minutes

Cooking time: 40 minutes

Servings: 4

Ingredients

- Two large potatoes
- One tablespoon of olive oil
- Salt to taste

Directions:

1. Peel the potatoes and cut them regularly
2. Preheat the Air fryer without oil at 180 ° C
3. Put the potatoes inside the Air fryer without oil for 25 minutes
4. Add salt to taste

Nutrition:

Calories: 234 Kcal / 100 gr

Proteins: 3.6gr / 100 gr

Fat: 11gr / 100 gr

Carbohydrates: 34gr / 100 gr

Glycemic Index IG (CG): 70 (23.8u)

Air Fryer Calzones

Preparation Time: 10 minutes

Cooking time: 35 minutes

Servings: 4

Ingredients

- One teaspoon oil

- One/4 cup finely cut purple onion (from 1 tiny onion)

- three ounces baby spinach leaves (about 3 cups)

- 1/3 cup lower-sodium spaghetti sauce

- 2 ounces sliced rotisserie pigeon breast (about 1/3 cup)

- 6 ounces recent ready grain dish dough

- 1 1/2 ounces pre-shredded part-skim cheese (about 5 Tbsp.)

- Cooking spray

Directions:

1. Heat oil in a very medium slippery frypan over medium-high. Add onion, and then

cook, sometimes stirring, till tender, 2 minutes. Add spinach; cowl and cook till limp, 1 1/2 minutes. Take away pan from heat; stir in spaghetti sauce and chicken.

2. Divide dough into four equal items.

3. Roll each bit on a gently floured surface into a 6-inch circle.

4. Place a quarter of the spinach mixture over 1/2 every dough process. Prime is every with a quarter of the cheese. Fold dough over filling to make half-moons, crimping edges to seal—coat calzones well with preparation spray.

5. Place calzones inside air fryer basket, and cook at 325°F till the dough is a golden brown, 12 minutes, turning calzones over once eight minutes.

Nutrition

Calories 348

Fat 12g

Sat fat 3g

Unsafe 7g

Protein 21g

Carbohydrate 44g

Fiber 5g

Sugars 3g

Added sugars 0g

Sodium 710mg

Calcium 21 DV

Potassium 3 DV

Crispy Air-Fried Onion Rings With Comeback Sauce

Preparation Time: 10 minutes

Cooking time: 35 minutes

Servings: 4

Ingredients

- 1/2 cup (about a pair of 1/8 oz.) general-purpose flour

- One teaspoon preserved paprika

- 1/2 teaspoon kosher salt, divided

- One giant egg

- One tablespoon water

- 1 cup grain panko (Japanese-style breadcrumbs)

- 1 (10-oz.) sweet onion, dig 1/2-in.-thick rounds and separated into rings

- Cooking spray

- 1/4 cup direct 1 Chronicles low-fat Greek food

- Two tablespoons canola mayo

- One tablespoon tomato ketchup

- One teaspoon metropolis mustard

- 1/4 teaspoon garlic powder

- 1/4 teaspoon paprika

Directions:

1. Stir along flour, preserved paprika, and 1/4 teaspoon of the salt in a very shallow dish. Gently beat egg and water in a very second shallow dish. Stir along with panko and remaining 1/4 teaspoon salt in a very third shallow dish. Dredge onion rings inside the flour mixture, shaking off excess. Dip in egg mixture, permitting any excess to drip off. Dredge in panko mixture, pressing to stick. Coat each side of onion rings well with preparation spray.

2. Put onion rings in a single layer inside air fryer basket, and cook in batches at 375°F till golden brown and tender on each side, 10 minutes, turning onion rings over

halfway through preparation. The cowl has stayed heat whereas practice is remaining onion rings.

3. Meanwhile, stir along with food, mayonnaise, ketchup, mustard, garlic powder, and paprika in a very tiny bowl till sleek. To serve, place VI to seven onion rings on every plate with a pair of tablespoons sauce.

Nutrition

Calories 174

Fat 5g

Sat fat 1g

Unsafe 3g

Protein 7g

Carbohydrate 25g

Fiber 3g

Sugars 5g

Added sugars 0g

Sodium 414mg

Calcium 4 % DV

Potassium 3 DV

Air-Fried Corn Dog Bites

Preparation Time: 10 minutes

Cooking time: 35 minutes

Servings: 4

Ingredients

- Two uncured all-beef hot dogs
- 12 craft sticks or bamboo skewers
- 1/2 cup (about a pair of 1/8 oz.) general-purpose flour
- Two giant eggs, gently crushed
- 1 1/2 cups crushed cornflakes cereal
- Cooking spray
- Eight teaspoons yellow mustard

Directions:

1. Slice every hot dog in lengthwise. Cut every one into three identical items. Insert a craft stick or use a bamboo skewer into one finish of every hot dog piece.

2. Place flour in a very shallow dish.

3. Place gently crushed eggs in a very second shallow dish. Place crushed cornflakes in a very third shallow dish.

4. Dredge hot dogs inside flour, shaking off excess. Dip in egg, permitting any excess to drip off. Dredge in cornflake crumbs, pressing to stick.

5. Lightly coat the air fryer basket is with preparation spray. Place VI corn dog bites in the basket; gently spray crack with preparation spray. Cook at 375°F till the coating is golden brown and crisp, 10 minutes, turning the corn dog bites over halfway through preparation. Repeat with remaining corn dog bites.

6. To serve, place three corn dog bites on every plate with a pair of teaspoons mustard, and serve instantly.

Nutrition

Calories 82

Fat 3g

Sat fat 1g

Unsafe 1g

Protein 5g

Carbohydrate 8g

Fiber 0g

Sugars 1g

Added sugars 0g

Sodium 179mg

Potassium 1/3 DV

Air-Fried Apple Chips

Preparation Time: 10 minutes

Cooking time: 40 minutes

Servings: 4

Ingredients

- 1 (8-oz.) apple (such as Fuji or Honey crisp)
- One teaspoon ground cinnamon
- Two teaspoons oil
- Cooking spray
- 1/4 cup plain I Chronicles low-fat Greek food
- One tablespoon almond butter
- One teaspoon honey

Directions:

1. Thinly slice apple on a mandoline. Place slices in an exceeding bowl with cinnamon and oil; toss to coat equally.

2. Coat air fryer basket as well with a change of state spray. Place seven to eight apple

slices in a single layer in a basket, cook at 375°F for twelve minutes, turn the pieces every four minutes, and rearrange portions to flatten them, as they'll move throughout the change of state method. Slices won't be fully crisped; however, they can still crisp upon cooling. Repeat with remaining apple slices.

3. While apple slices are cook, stir along with food, almond butter, and honey in an exceedingly tiny bowl till swish. To serve, place half dozen to eight apple slices on every plate with a little low small indefinite amount of dipping sauce.

Nutrition

Calories 104

Fat 3

Sat fat 1g

Unsatfat 2g

Protein 1g

Carbohydrate 17g

Fiber 3g

Sugars 4g

Added sugars 0g

Sodium 187mg

Calcium 3% DV

Potassium 4DV

Oregano And Sesame Sticks In The Air Fryer

Preparation Time: 10 minutes

Cooking time: 25 minutes

Servings: 8

Ingredients

- The egg that we have leftover to breach or one beaten egg

- Bread crumbs

- **Sesame**

- **Oregano**

Directions:

1. We bind the beaten egg with the breadcrumbs until it has dough.

2. We make balls and stretch them into sticks.

3. We go through sesame and oregano that we have linked on a plate.

4. We place in the basket of the Air fryer.

5. We select 20 minutes, 180 degrees.

6. We take out and serve.

Meatballs In Thermo Mix And Air Fryer

Preparation Time: 10 minutes

Cooking time: 35 minutes

Servings: 6

Ingredients

- 1 kg mixed minced meat
- One onion
- **One egg**
- One bunch of parsley
- Two cloves of garlic
- One lemon
- **Salt**
- Ground pepper
- Bread crumbs
- Extra virgin olive oil

Directions:

1. We put the minced meat in a bowl.

2. Salpimentamos.

3. In the Thermomix glass, we put the onion cut into quarters, the egg, the parsley, the garlic, and the lemon juice.

4. We select 7 seconds speed 5.

5. We dump the content in the minced meat and bind.

6. Add some breadcrumbs so that the meat loses some moisture.

7. We make the meatballs and go through the breadcrumbs.

8. Put the meatballs in batches in the basket of the air fryer and close the drawer.

9. We spray with oil.

10. We select 10 minutes of 200 degrees. We shake the basket and leave three more minutes.

11. We take out and make another batch of meatballs.

12. We serve

Fried Sardines In The Air Fryer

Preparation Time: 10 minutes

Cooking time: 30 minutes

Servings: 6

Ingredients

- 12 sardines

- Fishmeal

- **Salt**

- Extra virgin olive oil

Directions:

1. We clean the sardines, remove guts, and, if we want, the heads.

2. We put salt.

3. We pass the sardines for flour and shake well to remove the excess flour.

4. We put sardines, 4 in 4 or 6 in 6, in the air fryer basket, depending on the size, do not pile up.

5. We spray with oil.

6. We close the drawer with the basket inside.

7. We select between 180 to 200. Cook for about 10 minutes. Set a high temperature to make sardines crispy and golden.

8. At 10 minutes, we shake the sardines and check if they are ready or need a few more minutes.

9. When they are golden brown to our liking, we take out. We serve

10. Remember that there are no foods with the same color in this type of fryers when we fry the food submerged in oil.

Crab Balls In The Air Fryer

Preparation Time: 10 minutes

Cooking time: 30 minutes

Servings: 6

Ingredients

- 250 gr of crab sticks
- 50 gr of crusty bread without crust
- 50 gr of cream cheese
- 50 gr of milk
- **Salt**
- Whipped egg and breadcrumbs
- **Oil**

Directions:

1. We put all ingredients in the Thermomix glass.

2. We select 20 seconds speed 6.

3. We take the contents of the glass to a bowl and make small balls.

4. We pass the balls for breadcrumbs, then for beaten egg and again for breadcrumbs.

5. When we have them ready, we place them in the air fryer basket and spray with extra virgin olive oil.

6. We put the basket in the drawer and put it in the air fryer.

7. We select 160 degrees, 10 minutes. We shake the basket so that the balls change position.

8. We select 180 degrees, 10 minutes. We control, so they don't brown too much.

9. We serve

Mini Tatin Cake In The Air Fryer

Preparation Time: 10 minutes

Cooking time: 55 minutes

Servings: 4

Ingredients

- Two portions
- 100 gr flour
- 50 gr cold butter

- 25 ml Water

- One pinch Salt

- **1 Apple**

- Lemon juice

- 25 gr sugar

- 15 gr Butter

Directions:

1. The first thing to do will be the broken dough; we put the salt in the flour and the cold butter. We mix everything until it looks like sand.

2. Now we add the 25 ml of water and mix until obtaining a homogeneous mass that does not stick on the hands. We wrap it in transparent paper and reserve.

3. In a clay pot, we put the sugar and butter and let it melt and toast.

4. On the other hand, we descorazonamos and peel the apple, we will use the lemon juice to spread it, and that does not rust, we can also leave it in water with lemon.

5. When our sugar and butter are already golden, we put the apples on top. We will place them tightly, trying to cover the entire surface very well.

6. We leave the apples caramelizing for 15 to 20 minutes. We will control them.

7. Meanwhile, we stretched the dough. I made it with a rolling pin and using the baking paper. But you can do it as you find it more comfortable.

8. Once the apples are caramelized, we cover them with the broken dough. Cut what is leftover and adjust to the contour. We also puncture with a fork to give way to steam.

9. Preheat the fryer to 160 degrees, and put the cake for about 15 minutes.

10. After this time is ready, we will let it sit at room temperature to remove it quickly. We pass a knife around the edges and turn around. Enjoy!!

Rabas Is A Hot Air Fryer

Preparation Time: 10 minutes

Cooking time: 35 minutes

Servings: 4

Ingredients

- 16 rabas

- **One egg**

- Bread crumbs

- Condiments: salt, pepper, sweet paprika

Directions:

1. In my case, they were frozen, so I put them in hot water, and they boil for 2 minutes.

2. Remove and dry well.

3. Beat the egg and season to taste. I put salt, pepper, and sweet paprika—place in the egg.

4. Bread with breadcrumbs. Place in sticks.

5. Place in the fryer for 5 minutes at 160 degrees. Remove

6. Spray with fritolin and place five more minutes at 200 degrees.

Banana Split

Preparation Time: 15 minutes

Cooking Time: 14 minutes

Servings: 8

Ingredients:

- Three tablespoons coconut oil

- 1 cup panko breadcrumbs

- ½ cup of cornflour

- Two eggs

- Four bananas, peeled and halved lengthwise

- Three tablespoons sugar

- ¼ teaspoon ground cinnamon

- Two tablespoons walnuts, chopped

Directions:

1. In a medium skillet, melt the coconut oil over medium heat and cook breadcrumbs

for about 3-4 minutes or until golden browned and crumbled, stirring continuously.

2. Transfer the breadcrumbs into a shallow bowl and set aside to cool.

3. In a second bowl, place the cornflour.

4. In a third bowl, whisk the eggs.

5. Coat the banana slices with flour, dip into eggs, and finally coat evenly with the breadcrumbs.

6. In a small bowl, mix the sugar and cinnamon.

7. Press "Power Button" of Air Fry Oven and turn the dial to select the "Air Fry" mode.

8. Press the Time button and again turn the dial to set the cooking time to 10 minutes.

9. Now push the Temp button and rotate the dial to set the temperature at 280 degrees F.

10. Press the "Start/Pause" button to start.

11. When the unit beeps to show that it is preheated, open the lid.

12. Arrange the banana slices in "Air Fry Basket" and sprinkle with cinnamon sugar.

13. Insert the basket in the oven.

14. Transfer the banana slices onto plates to cool slightly

15. Sprinkle with chopped walnuts and serve.

Nutrition:

Calories 216

Total Fat 8.8g

Saturated Fat 5.3 g

Cholesterol 41 mg

Sodium 16 mg

Total Carbs 26 g

Fiber 2.3 g

Sugar 11.9 g

Protein 3.4 g

Crispy Banana Slices

Preparation Time: 15 minutes

Cooking Time: 15 minutes

Servings: 8

Ingredients:

- Four medium ripe bananas, peeled

- 1/3 cup rice flour, divided

- Two tablespoons all-purpose flour

- Two tablespoons cornflour

- Two tablespoons desiccated coconut

- ½ teaspoon baking powder

- ½ teaspoon ground cardamom

- Pinch of salt

- Water, as required

- ¼ cup sesame seeds

Directions:

1. In a shallow bowl, mix two tablespoons of rice flour, all-purpose flour, cornflour, coconut, baking powder, cardamom, and salt.

2. Gradually, add the water and mix until a thick and smooth mixture forms.

3. In a second bowl, place the remaining rice flour.

4. In a third bowl, add the sesame seeds.

5. Cut each banana into half and then cut each half into two pieces lengthwise.

6. Dip the banana slices into the coconut mixture and then coat with the remaining rice flour, followed by the sesame seeds.

7. Press "Power Button" of Air Fry Oven and turn the dial to select the "Air Fry" mode.

8. Press the Time button and again turn the dial to set the cooking time to 15 minutes.

9. Now push the Temp button and rotate the dial to set the temperature at 390 degrees F.

10.   Press the "Start/Pause" button to start.

11.   When the unit beeps to show that it is preheated, open the lid.

12.   Arrange the banana slices in "Air Fry Basket" and insert it in the oven.

13.   Transfer the banana slices onto plates to cool slightly

14.   Transfer the banana slices onto plates to cool slightly before serving.

Nutrition:

Calories 121

Total Fat 3 g

Saturated Fat 0.8g

Cholesterol 0 mg

Sodium 21 mg

Total Carbs 23.1 g

Fiber 2.6 g

Sugar 7.3 g

Protein 2.2 g

Pineapple Bites

Preparation Time: 10 minutes

Cooking Time: 10 minutes

Servings: 4

Ingredients:

For Pineapple Sticks:

- ½ of pineapple

- ¼ cup desiccated coconut

For Yogurt Dip:

- One tablespoon fresh mint leaves, minced

- 1 cup vanilla yogurt

Directions:

1. Remove the outer skin of the pineapple and cut into long 1-2 inch thick sticks.

2. In a shallow dish, place the coconut.

3. Coat the pineapple sticks with coconut evenly.

4. Press "Power Button" of Air Fry Oven and turn the dial to select the "Air Fry" mode.

5. Press the Time button and again turn the dial to set the cooking time to 10 minutes.

6. Now push the Temp button and rotate the dial to set the temperature at 390 degrees F.

7. Press the "Start/Pause" button to start.

8. When the unit beeps to show that it is preheated, open the lid.

9. Arrange the pineapple sticks in a lightly greased "Air Fry Basket" and insert it in the oven.

10. Meanwhile, for a dip in a bowl, mix mint and yogurt.

11. Serve pineapple sticks with yogurt dip.

Nutrition:

Calories 124

Total Fat 2.6 g

Saturated Fat 21 g

Cholesterol 4 mg

Sodium 46 mg

Total Carbs 21.6 g

Fiber 2.3 g

Sugar 16.9 g

Protein 4.4 g

Cheesecake Bites

Preparation Time: 20 minutes

Cooking Time: 2 minutes

Servings: 12

Ingredients:

- 8 oz. cream cheese, softened

- ½ cup plus two tablespoons sugar, divided

- Four tablespoons heavy cream, divided

- ½ teaspoon vanilla extract

- ½ cup almond flour

Directions:

1. In a stand mixer bowl, fitted with the paddle attachment, add the cream cheese, ½ cup of sugar, two tablespoons of heavy cream, and vanilla extract and beat until smooth.

2. With a scooper, scoop the mixture onto a parchment paper-lined baking pan.

3. Freeze for about 30 minutes or until firm.

4. In a small bowl, place the remaining cream.

5. In another small bowl, add the almond flour and the remaining sugar and mix well.

6. Dip each cheesecake bite in cream and then coat with the flour mixture.

7. Press "Power Button" of Air Fry Oven and turn the dial to select the "Air Fry" mode.

8. Press the Time button and again turn the dial to set the cooking time to 2 minutes.

9. Now push the Temp button and rotate the dial to set the temperature at 300 degrees F.

10. Press the "Start/Pause" button to start.

11. When the unit beeps to show that it is preheated, open the lid.

12. Arrange the pan in "Air Fry Basket" and insert it in the oven.

13. Serve warm.

Nutrition:

Calories 149

Total Fat 10.7 g

Saturated Fat 5.5 g

Cholesterol 28 mg

Sodium 60 mg

Total Carbs 11.7 g

Fiber 0.5 g

Sugar 10.1 g

Protein 2.5 g